A POWERHOUSE OF PRAISE!

"Full of potentially life-saving knowledge....The book's comprehensiveness, its well-organized contents, and its absence of confusing medical terminology make it particularly useful."
— *Natural Health*

"Easy to digest....Rosenfeld's levelheaded, straightforward, informative style will reassure many patients."
— *Publishers Weekly*

"The real value of this book is the nifty guide at the end of each chapter that outlines 'What to insist on if you have...(fill in the disease.)'"

— *Palm Beach Post*

"Dr. Rosenfeld fills a heartfelt need....Women may find the book particularly useful."

— *Bookloons*

Live Now, Age Later

Dr. Rosenfeld's Guide to Alternative Medicine

Doctor, What Should I Eat?

The Best Treatment

Symptoms

Modern Prevention

Second Opinion

The Complete Medical Exam

The Electrocardiogram and
Chest X-ray in Diseases
of the Heart